Table of Contents

The Impact of Allergies on Sleep Quality and Strategies for Creating a Healthy Sleeping Environment

Factors Contributing to Worsening Allergies at Night

1. Introduction to Allergies and Allergic Reactions

Due to this, man experiences various side-effects such as sinuses, itchy skin, rashes, skin hives, stomach discomfort, sudden inflammations, changes in mood, or mental state. Moreover, the intensity and severity of an allergic attack are often determined by the individual's health and lifestyle habits, treatment or medication, nutrition, environmental situation, genetics, etc. Depending on the severity of your allergies, symptoms could differ from person to person such as itchy or tearing eyes, sinus pressure, throat irritation, sneezing, and chest tightness, and for people with asthma, it is important to ensure that during allergic episodes their inhaler is close by. Furthermore, sometimes, the intensity and seriousness of a person's allergic symptoms can escalate or worsen at night, and medical researchers and allergists have examined the potential factors or causes for this development and have explained the underlying reasons associated with it.

The human body's immune system is complex and extremely sensitive, and therefore often susceptible to severe reactions when exposed to specific allergens. Allergies refer to an abnormal, vigorous reaction of a person's immunity in response to a foreign substance such as food, pet dander, pollen, dust, and the likes. When an individual experiences an allergic attack, his or her immune system mistakenly associates a seemingly mild substance or food particle with a potential threat by responding in a variety of ways to ensure that that threat is neutralized.

2. Circadian Rhythms and Allergy Symptoms

Research has shown that the body's immune system fluctuates, suggesting the time of day allergens are taken can influence a mature immune system's response. According to the study, a mature adult takes longer to develop allergies than a child or elderly individual. The more mature the immune system, the less likely different blood cells travel to the lungs, release mucus, and fluids in response to allergies. Individual white blood cells display different superficial proteins at different times of the day. According to researchers, this could be linked to a better immune response in the morning; for example, specific immune cells merge to produce an anti-inflammatory drug because certain gene switches are activated. According to researchers, symptoms vary throughout the day for individuals with allergies, asthma, and other fungal diseases. A runny nose, for example, typically worsens between midnight and 4 AM, and coughing or wheezing worsens between 3 and 4 AM.

Substantial evidence exists corroborating the relationship between your body's internal clock and allergy symptoms. Scientists argue that our "body clock" influences allergic responses, meaning your allergy symptoms may worsen in the evening and at night. Circadian rhythms are behavioral, physical, and mental changes following a 24-hour cycle, such as your body setting its wake and sleep schedule according to the light outside. The suprachiasmatic nucleus

– a small group of nerve cells in the hypothalamus –
controls your body's internal clock. Time-giving cells
control functions that include temperature, hormone
secretion, and cell production. All cells carry these clocks,
much like they carry your genes. It is believed allergies are
worse in the evening and at night because your body tends
to become more sensitive, boosts its chemical-producing
bile, and makes miniature alarms go off, like mast cells,
that direct certain parts of your body to react.

2.1. Understanding the Body's Internal Clock

The environmental time cues are called the Zeitgebers, the most critical being the light/dark cycle, to which the body can respond either directly to the light perception or indirectly. Although the suprachiasmatic nuclei in the brain, that contain thousands of clock neurons, are mostly responsible to generate the light patterns throughout the whole body, a lot of cells have their own molecular clock machinery that is managed by the suprachiasmatic nuclei in response to light. When this inner clock is disturbed, the body does not work properly, or health issues appear, with diseases such as sleep disorders, mental health problems, obesity, diabetes, depression, bipolar disorder, and various types of cancer, where the time and the mode of the disruption influence the type of pathology.

The body keeps its own schedule with the help of the internal clock, adhering to the circadian rhythms. This cycle regulates various body aspects, such as the release of hormones and body temperature, and the internal clock is mostly influenced by the environment but also by genetics, age, and health status. This rhythm is activated by the so-called clock genes that, when active, produce proteins that prevent genes from becoming active. With time, the concentration of these proteins begins to drop and new ones are no longer produced, and the genes are no longer blocked and become active. Once this happens, genes instruct the body to produce new proteins that stop the genes from functioning. There are whole sets of genes that help the maintenance of circadian rhythms in various molecular pathways.

2.2. Impact of Circadian Rhythms on Allergic Responses

In allergic diseases, including eosinophilic diseases, the secretion of proteins and chemicals from eosinophils is associated with driving allergic inflammations. Previous work has demonstrated that in humans and in animal models of allergies, the allergic response can be subject to what are called diurnal variations. These diurnal variations are variations that occur based on the time of day and predict that allergic responses will be at their worst at night and early in the morning. This has been found in both allergic rhinitis, or 'hay fever,' where symptoms of nasal congestion, eye itch, and sneezing can drive many patients to seek medical relief, and in eosinophilic diseases like eosinophilic esophagitis (EoE) where allergic inflammation causes difficulty swallowing, initially in infants, until food occasionally sticks and causes chest pain, vomiting, inability to eat, and occasionally damage to the esophagus.

The master clock in the brain regulates both sleep-wake patterns as well as other biological patterns, such as body temperature, blood pressure, and hormone levels. Based on this master clock, every cell in the body has a miniature clock, and together, they control and anticipate key biochemical and signaling activities centered on particular times of the day. Work in research laboratories worldwide has revealed that circadian clocks influence not only the immune systems, but also the severity and timing of symptoms that are most closely linked to one type of white blood cell, the eosinophil.

3. Indoor Allergens and Nighttime Exposure

At any time of the day, it is possible to be exposed to numerous allergens, be it indoors, outdoors, or at work. Although exposure to allergens is often multifactorial, the main allergens present indoors are animal dander, dust mite, cockroach, mold and fungi spores, as well as particulate matter. These are present in the living environment as feeding sites for cockroaches or their waste, dander from animals that live with us or are in the building, or inorganic or organic material that accumulates as part of the human environment. Cases of occupational exposure are typically limited to certain professions that deal with animals or textiles. One of the most powerful stimuli for allergic reactions is the allergy season, or symptomotypes or responses to presentation. In another type of exposure, an individual is exposed to an allergen during the day, which could result in a worsening of health symptoms in the evening or overnight. It is hypothesized that during the day, the individual is exposed to allergens in their everyday routine or life and experiences a response at the time when the responses normally peak or get worse. The endogenous circadian rhythm is based on a 24-hour pattern with regular time intervals of activity and rest, both of which are recurrent.

While commonplace, the presence of these allergens indoors suggests that many people are at least occasionally exposed to them. It is not known whether the nighttime worsening is a direct result of a stronger reaction to these allergens, but exposure to these allergens may lead to a build-up of sensitivity over the course of the day or sensitize an individual in the evening, thereby making them more sensitive in the morning. There might also be a combined effect of being exposed to several allergens all day long. Nevertheless, the general aim of this chapter is to explore the relationship between indoor allergens and nighttime exposure. It will describe in more detail the common indoor allergens, particularly those that are likely to create nighttime disruption, and discuss the mechanisms by which these might contribute to nighttime allergies, which we will refer to as nocturnal allergies.

3.1. Common Indoor Allergens

Moisture, heat, darkness, and other external factors can cause dust mites to multiply, with the majority of the activity. In many beds, pillows, mattresses, and bedding encasements, a portion between the 100,000 and 10 million dust mites Marco Sterk lives. For highly sensitive people, as few as ten mites can generate symptoms. Dust mites are often found in carpets, upholstery, and the like. If cat allergen is a key factor in a person's allergic reaction, and the goal is to reduce the recurrence of cat viewing, then probably so far as removing the floors, it is feasible where a few of the feasible as well as very effective treatments. A clinic will help in increasing airflow, and as a consequence, air temperatures, could be applied to relieve respiratory symptoms and dyspnea through this drug. It was this same approach that helped in reducing the somewhat deceptive costs.

Common Indoor Allergens: House dust mites, animal dander, skin particles, cockroaches, and fungi are only a few examples of pests. According to Emert's rating in Reading, Massachusetts, the following are the most common allergy by geographic region as well as United States primary urban areas: a. Ragweed b. Trees, including Juniper, Cedar Elm, Birch, and Maple c. Grasses d. Mold and Yeast e. Dust Mites on Pediatrician

There are a variety of allergens found throughout indoor spaces that may bring about symptoms and health problems among those with allergies and for those who are sensitive to certain irritants. The most common indoor allergens are the proteins in pet hair, dander, skin wrinkling, and other irritants. These irritants, which amount to less than 10 microns, penetrate the internal environment and ultimately lead to the worsening of allergy conditions, such as waking up at night due to itching, respiratory congestion, and chronic coughing.

3.2. Sources of Indoor Allergens at Night

With the exception of dust mites, who generally don't leave their mattresses when people are sleeping in their beds, these allergen sources represent places people frequently occupy at night, during times when the building is essentially sealed up to provide the most comfort or energy. Bedding materials are likely extensive sources of house dust mites unless they are air permeable and of little interest to such organisms, or have been subjected to special cleaning that removes mites. The skin particles that provide food for mites, and the dead mites and their excrement, are likely to accumulate on and within fabrics. Cockroach and fungus particles are also larger than most dust mite particles are and are likely to be contacted or directly inhaled if they are present in an area of activity. Cockroach body parts, in particular, have been found to settle out of the air onto the sleeping tenant. Therefore, mattresses, bedding, and linens which gain the attention of dust mites, cockroaches, and fungus provide a likely source of exposure to indoor pest and fungal allergens at night when people are immersed in these materials. Some of these places can also harbor mold (fungus) in addition to living and dead dust mites, their eggs, and their cast skins.

Several indoor allergens come from multiple sources. Pollen is a widely known environmental allergen, but other potential sources of indoor allergens appear to be the biggest contributor of allergy symptoms at night. The most common indoor allergens originate either from within the indoor environment or from outdoors. House dust mites are often considered indoor allergens, since the aged females within their communities release a substantial number of allergen-containing particles. Fungus can be both an indoor and an outdoor allergen. Cockroaches commonly infest the home and are another source of indoor allergens. All of these potential sources of allergens thrive in warm moist environments and all release allergens which can result in the continuous presence of airborne particles that are likely to be inhaled by occupants.

4. Air Quality and Humidity Levels in Bedrooms

Air consists of moisture and air - the temperature the air can hold water vapor is reported as a relative humidity (RH) value. Based on the relative humidity, the air can either be too dry, typical of our winter-time homes, causing dry skin, stuffy noses, dry throats, and eyes, or too moist, contributing to the growth of mold, dust mites, and related reactions. A healthy home environment should have between 35 - 50% relative humidity throughout all rooms of the house. Since the average person spends approximately 8 hours sleeping in the bedroom, adjusting the moisture levels in that room to 35 - 50% should reduce symptoms of allergy caused by dust and mold these little critters love to call their home. "For the bed, materials that are allergen-proof or encased in allergen-proof covers are recommended," said Myerson.

Poor air quality may be making your allergy symptoms worse overnight. As dust and other allergy-provoking particles, such as pollen, mold, animal dander, and dust mites, accumulate in the air, they can settle in the bedroom where you spend one-third of your life. "The concentration of allergens in the air in room spaces is based on the rate of production and accumulation of the allergen, and on the ventilation designed to dilute and remove the allergen from the room," said Dr. Sally Myerson, director of the division of allergy and clinical immunology at the UMDNJ-New Jersey Medical School in Newark. "Through the magic

of gravity, most of these allergens will end up on the floor
and other surfaces in the room where they remain ready to
be kicked back up into the air to be inhaled by room
occupants or visitors."

4.1. Effects of Poor Air Quality on Allergies

The analysis of why other diseases - similar to those of the upper and lower phrasal tract - worsen at night can also be investigated. In this work, we aimed to highlight the aforementioned aspects about allergic symptoms worsened by night as further support. We report some mechanisms that reinforce the overlap among the aforementioned pathologies, focusing our attention on allergic symptoms. This manuscript must also teach readers to look for the etiological causal factors: not the allergic substances nor the technical barrier devices, but the environmental drivers or agents for a 24hr susceptible to non-delayed allergic disease, e.g. inflammation.

Poor air quality, in general, affects allergy symptoms. Inhabiting environments with air-contaminating particles, gases, textiles, insufficient ventilation, and stuffed belongings tend to experience worsening allergy symptoms. These conditions afflict people who spend long periods sick or need to be nursed, as they spend much time in their gerific, biocontaminated environments. In many cases, those affected by airborne-allergen-driven inflammatory diseases manifest allergic symptoms only in certain periods, such as the night. Respirators, allergologists, meteorologists, and even allergenimeric immunologists will find it interesting as they experience - during their night shift - a worsening of their breathing capacity when they enter a "pressurized" or polluted environment in which they cannot circulate.

4.2. Optimal Humidity Levels for Allergy Relief

In addition to bedroom humidity level, the climate in which you live has an impact on the quantity of dust mites in your environment. Optimal conditions for dust mite proliferation are 20°C and 70 percent relative humidity, according to Australian researchers. In the United States, the greatest humidity levels are seen in the southeastern portion of the nation, while the northeastern and western areas have drier climates. Low TrueSteamTM asthma & allergy relief steam humidifiers are simple to use and control, and they are a worthwhile investment in your home. A steam humidifier that connects to your home's climate monitor/thermostat can help keep your home's air quality within a safe range, which can help you tackle morning congestion brought on by dry, cooler air.

A major cause of nighttime allergy symptoms is dry air. In fact, a study published in the journal Clinical & Experimental Allergy showed that allergens get easily dispersed in the air when humidity levels remain low. According to a review published in the Journal of Allergy and Clinical Immunology in 2012, encasing bedding, pillows, and mattresses in allergy-proof covers helps to mitigate nighttime allergy triggers, such as dust mites. What's more, a 2014 issue of the journal Human & Experimental Toxicology evaluated over 202,000 asthma sufferers in 15 countries and discovered that a 70.5% relative humidity level discouraged the growth of dust mites and molds. To ensure a consistent relative humidity level in your bedroom, and, as a result, reduce the activities of these airborne allergens, consider investing in a high-quality humidifier to make it simple to breathe around bedtime. A relative humidity range encompassing 40 to 50 percent is considered to be optimal for decreasing airborne allergen exposure in humans.

5. Sleep Disruption and Allergy Symptoms

In discussing the factors contributing to worsening allergies at night, it becomes apparent to the reader that sleep disruption and allergy symptoms are closely intertwined. Misery at bedtime and nasal congestion upon waking are not only common complaints and allergen-associated symptoms, but they also reveal a critical connection between allergies and sleep. This bidirectional relationship is well-documented in both objective and subjective research. People with allergic rhinitis experience nocturnal symptoms and are subsequently more tired and fatigued than those without allergies. Research has also shown that sleep disruption is far worse when allergy symptoms are present, and strong evidence suggests that allergic rhinitis contributes significantly to the burden of sleep-disordered breathing. Most importantly, certain conclusions can be drawn about the connections between sleep and allergic rhinitis: allergies make it hard to get to sleep, and once they are asleep, allergies make it difficult to maintain sleep quality. This suggests that rhinitis-induced sleep disruption is separate from allergy-provoked upper airway resistance or sleep-disordered breathing, which tend to result in an awakening, rather than difficulty falling asleep. If allergies can cause insomnia, what purpose does oppressing sleep serve for the body? In order to prevent allergens such as dust mites from causing inflammation in nasal and pulmonary tissues, increased alertness during periods of natural allergen re-exposure and environmental exposure would be a wise defensive mechanism. For individuals who are allergic to common household allergens, becoming more vigilant at dusk and throughout the night would certainly be advantageous to their health. At the same time, our ability to become sleepy and fall asleep can also cause rhinitis symptoms to worsen, making it more difficult to sleep and stay asleep. A terrible cycle of feelings arises between allergies and snooze, with one causing the other to deteriorate until a proper environment is established.

The journal article "Factors Contributing to Worsening Allergies at Night" considers several factors that can cause allergy symptoms to worsen at night. The article describes allergy symptoms and factors that cause them to be worse at night for different types of allergies. A range of allergy medications and treatments are also discussed to aid individuals in modifying their behavior, help healthcare professionals and researchers in their work, and enhance the potential benefit of drugs or treatments that may become available in the future.

5.1. Bidirectional Relationship between Allergies and Sleep

Empiric evidence reveals that nasal resistance and thus nose fruit symptoms are much greater during rapid eye movement (REM) sleep rather than slow wave or deep slow wave sleep. Nasal resistance is also elevated during nonrapid eye movement (NREM) phase changes to REM. A stressful life event, if experienced in a typical dimension of psychological distress, can exacerbate allergy symptoms for at least a few days and as long as six weeks. A stressor that causes several physiologic changes and is associated with an increase in nocturnal sympathetic activity comprises sleep disruption.

Allergies and sleep: More than just being 'unpleasant,' many individuals feel that regular sleep disruptions qualify as something that warrants seeking professional advice. Many allergy sufferers find that symptoms routinely, and typically at a specific time of night or morning, force them to wake up. That being said, allergic sensitization and actual allergic diseases, like allergic rhinitis, sinus diseases, asthma, eczema, and anaphylactic problems must be considered when discussing 'allergy.' Questions abound as to whether or not these diseases have a direct causal role in sleep problems. Regardless of concurrent medical problems, it is also possible that these symptoms can be triggered or worsened by disturbances in sleep.

5.2. Strategies to Improve Sleep Quality for Allergy Sufferers

Improving the sleep environment: Ideally, the sleep environment should be kept allergy-free. High-quality mattresses and pillowcases can prevent allergens from entering them. The bedroom should also be protected from potential sources of allergens (e.g., by sealing the windows or using an air filter). Engaging in a set of actions may also make it easier for cleaning to be completed with low effort, such as not having carpets and blinds or other accessories that accumulate dust mites. Puffing up the pillows or shaking the duvet/quilt outside could spread the mites into the air and exacerbate the allergies. Mattresses and pillows often accumulate high levels of dust mites. Hence, they should be dusted, the sheets should be vacuumed, and the bedding should be washed in hot water to kill any dust mites. Pet allergens could potentially be found all over the house, such as pets' lowers, beds, and floors. District heaters and indiscriminate air filters can reduce the dispersion of allergens in the house, leading to an improved environment for people with pet allergies.

Allergies and their symptoms can be especially difficult to cope with at night. In addition to seasonal allergies, such as hay fever, many people with dust mite allergies or pet allergies find that their symptoms worsen during and after sleep. These individuals sometimes wake up because of the symptoms and find it hard to go back to sleep. For others, their sleep may be constantly disrupted during the night by their symptoms. While the development of new treatments specifically targeting these nocturnal symptoms is needed, there are some strategies that may help allergy sufferers get better sleep.

Strategies to improve sleep quality for people with allergies

6. Medication Timing and Efficacy

The optimal time for each type of medication will vary as well. Here are just a few examples. Oral antihistamines typically should be taken in the morning, as the drowsiness produced by many of these drugs will have worn off by nightfall, leaving you more alert throughout the day. Antihistamine eye drops and decongestant nasal sprays can also help alleviate symptoms that make it difficult to sleep if taken in the daytime. Corticosteroid nasal sprays are typically the best option for bedtime use, as they can take two or three days to reach full effectiveness. Be sure to ask your physician for the best timing for your specific medication choices.

No matter the contributing factors for worsening allergies at night, the goal of most is to be able to treat and manage these symptoms so you can get a good night's rest. One of the first lines of defense for allergies is allergy medications. There are a wide variety of allergy medications available, including over-the-counter and prescription medication. The type of medication that will work best for you can vary from person to person. Some medication options include antihistamines, corticosteroids, decongestants, leukotriene modifiers, and immunomodulators (medications that suppress your immune system and are typically used for those with chronic allergies that do not respond to other treatments). Medication can be taken orally, by injection, or through an inhaler. Various forms such as pills, chewable tablets, nasal sprays, or eye drops are also available.

6.1. Types of Allergy Medications

Nasal sprays are the most popular type of corticosteroids used for the treatment of allergies, especially when nasal congestion is a big problem. Corticosteroids help fight the inflammation caused by airborne irritants. Even though the nose spray is aimed at the sinuses, low levels of the drug reach the back of the throat, which is why these are the best allergy drugs to help with asthma and throat issues. Many medical professionals recommend using a decongestant as part of the treatment for nighttime allergies. This over-the-counter medication shrinks the blood vessels in the nasal passages to open up airways. Unlike some of the medications named above, a decongestant can be taken alone, although you should always ask a doctor about combination therapy for allergy treatment. These medications also come as a topical treatment that can help as a quick solution for sinus issues. However, patients can only use these medications for an average of three days to avoid the rebound effect, a worsening of symptoms when use is stopped.

When it comes to treating nighttime allergies, doctors prefer using a combination of two types of allergy medications: antihistamines and corticosteroids. Antihistamines reduce the production of histamine, a chemical produced when the body is exposed to an allergen or irritant like pet dander, pollen, or dust. This drug is a popular treatment for itchy, watery eyes, sneezing, hives, and a runny nose. While antihistamines are most commonly used as a tablet or liquid, medical professionals can also recommend an over-the-counter (OTC) or prescription eye drop for those affected by watery, itchy eyes.

6.2. Optimal Timing for Allergy Medication Administration

The timing of taking allergy medication may be less important for nasal congestion as it can recover faster if nasal steroids and mast cell stabilizers are used during the day and are continued at night. However, compliance may be an issue, especially if daytime nasal congestion is tolerable. If antihistamines are only taken during the day, it is less effective in controlling nighttime nasal congestion. Corticosteroid injections and Leukotriene Receptor Antagonists (LTRAs) are considered problematic when it comes to nighttime use because they can cause insomnia. Meta-analyses of clinical trials have shown that taking LTRAs in the evening improves lung volumes in subjects with nocturnal asthma. INCSs can be started the day with no added benefit for night symptoms if taking a second dose in the evening. However, a greater effect is observed when inhaled Fluticasone is taken every morning and evening. Mast cell stabilizers may be effective if used every 12 hours for allergic rhinitis symptoms, but evidence regarding effectiveness when only used in the morning is lacking.

The optimal timing for the administration of allergy medication largely depends on the agent chosen. Antihistamines, both first- and second-generations, should ideally be taken before bedtime to allow enough time for the medication's peak effects to provide relief. Other agents, such as intranasal corticosteroid sprays and leukotriene receptor antagonists (LTRAs), can be effective when taken in the morning and evening for reduction of nighttime symptoms. Any of these medications can be taken as needed during the day or night for greater symptom relief if severe symptoms persist.

7. Conclusion and Recommendations for Managing Nighttime Allergies

This interest in the patients' lifestyle, hygiene, and weight reflects concerns about allergen control in the environment. Far from being just a guide for managing or predicting common allergies, this article took into account scientific studies and patients' experiences to discuss the trajectory of common allergies in three different aspects: in the present, in the past, and even in the future.

Results showed that better knowledge of night allergies correlates with better sleep quality, showing the relevance of the night symptom management. After an accurate analysis of our topics, when allergies flare up at night, we suggest: placing a HEPA-filter air cleaning device in your bedroom to filter pollen, use special pet sheets that decrease pet hair and dander; clean your bed sheets and change your pillowcase often to get rid of dust mites; take a shower at night to rinse off any remaining pollen that might be lingering in your hair or skin.

In conclusion, good strategies to prevent or alleviate nighttime allergy symptoms depend on the chronotype and are worth tailoring to individual clinical characteristics. In the meantime, considering the nose occlusion situation is also a research point.

In conclusion, night worsens allergies due to diverse factors, including hormonal fluctuations, circadian rhythms, air pollutants, and amendments in personal behavior. To reduce or prevent allergic symptoms at night might also rely on the type of allergic disease. In patients with allergic rhinitis, for instance, simple actions like using air purifiers and avoiding pet allergens might help make sleep hours free from symptoms.

The Impact of Allergies on Sleep Quality and Strategies for Creating a Healthy Sleeping Environment

1. Introduction to Allergies and Sleep

Most individuals develop some kind of allergy at some point in their lives, and up to 30 percent of people worldwide have allergic rhinitis. The essay will concentrate on the causes behind allergic sleep disturbances because of the work of allergic rhinitis. People commonly encounter air quality deficiencies due to viruses or fungal spores. People who already have allergies would encounter a significant burden when encountering these conditions because their immune systems have already been primed to overreact to these substances. Another possible cause of disrupted sleep is the intensity of high-allergen-level sleeping environments. The bedroom, like any other space, can be an allergy-friendly habitat when designed effectively. Ultimately, the bedroom area of any house is a sanctuary where one should be able to relax, refresh, recharge, and get a decent night's sleep. Overcoming allergies in the bedroom may aid in maintaining it as a clean space.

Allergies are a natural defense mechanism of the immune system and are often controllable. Inadequate sleep quality is a common condition that is disturbing people's quality of life. People who have allergies, such as hay fever and other allergic rhinitis, may experience setbacks and challenges in obtaining good sleep. Nasal obstruction and congestion, as well as sneezing, itching, and postnasal drainage, will interfere with a person's ability to sleep or remain sleeping. This essay discusses the pathophysiology of diseases and mechanistic evidence predicting the relationship between allergies and inadequate sleep, as well as coping techniques to help people get cleaner, healthier sleep.

1.1. Understanding Allergies

House-dust mites, with their allergen-filled droppings, pollens from grass, trees and weeds, pet dander, insect wastes, and other things all contribute to allergic reactions. Additionally, there is a link between poor sleep and allergic responses. Allergies of the nose or throat, which are exacerbated by exposure to house dust mites, result in almost nine out of ten people reporting a flare-up of their symptoms at night. Pollen allergies, pet allergies, and animal allergies cause sleeping difficulties in more than two-thirds of sinusitis patients because their irritating sinus symptoms are more pronounced during the day and evening. Naturopathic treatment for allergic patients was an important benefit of an expensive study conducted in the United States. Configuring the inside of the houses was one of the suggestions, which was given to this study. There are many strategies to make your sleeping environment free of allergies.

While allergies are widespread, many individuals are unfamiliar with the source of their discomfort. Our immune system defends the body against bacteria, viruses, and other pathogenic agents that may upset our health. The human immune system makes the mistake of attacking a drug, a type of food, or even a foreign substance as if it were seeking to harm the body in the event of an allergic response. These materials, which can trigger allergic reactions, are referred to as allergens. Highlands, animal dander, insect wastes, dust particles, pollen, and food are all common allergens. Allergic responses differ from individual to individual, and in general, they can be acute or chronic. Difficulties in smelling or breathing, coughing, eye and nose distress, hives, and rashes are all possible symptoms of an allergic response.

2. The Relationship Between Allergies and Sleep

Sleep and allergies can interact in a variety of ways. Studies show that having allergic rhinitis can double the chances of developing a sleep disorder. Female rhinitis sufferers report waking up more frequently and having a harder time falling asleep than men. Allergic rhinitis can interfere with sleep even if symptoms don't surface until late in the night. Fortunately, there are ways to manage allergies and help build a healthier sleep environment. By identifying what triggers your allergies, it's possible to reduce exposure to them. One such strategy is to keep pets out of the bedroom, as pet dander is a common allergen. You may also consider using a vacuum with a HEPA filter to remove allergen particles from the surfaces of your home.

Allergies and sleep are closely intertwined – allergies can cause poor-quality sleep and a lack of sleep can exacerbate an allergic reaction. Allergens are proteins from things like pet dander, mold spores, and dust mites. They are microscopic, lightweight, and travel through the air. Inhaling them can cause a variety of symptoms including sneezing, sniffling, and coughing. Common allergens that impact sleep include dust mites, pollen, mold, pet dander, and perfumes. Allergy symptoms caused by the release of histamine can impact quality sleep. Individuals who report feeling sleepy have a lower quality of life than those who are able to get at least seven hours of sleep a night. Inadequate sleep caused by allergies can affect mood, memory, and decision making. Over time, it can lead to a variety of health conditions.

2.1. Common Allergens Affecting Sleep

Many allergens can detrimentally influence sleep. Here, we show an overview of certain typical allergens as well as particular allergens' effects on various people. Dust mites are the most common indoor allergen. People inhale the body parts (fecal and decaying matter) of dust mites, which are consumed by house dust mite allergens that are released into the air when they roll around in bed, sit on a sofa, or walk on the carpeted floor in massive amounts. Symptoms: Unexpected sneezing, itchy eyes, or a runny nose. Strategies for getting rid of dust mites include utilizing machine-washable pillows, mattress coverings, blankets, and curtains. It is suggested that you wash your bedsheets and covers in hot water throughout the week (preferably 130°F or 54°C) to eliminate allergens.

Allergens can have a substantial impact on sleep. As the body rests and recovers during sleep, it becomes more susceptible to allergens, leading to difficulties. When asthma patients were surveyed about their concomitant symptoms, over 40 percent of respondents said that allergies induced wheezing at night. About 3 in 4 persons with perennial allergic rhinitis have disrupted sleep and diminished cognitive capacity due to illnesses. Individuals with food allergies have a higher chance of developing obstructive sleep-disordered breathing in addition to these two significant medical concerns. Obstructive sleep disorder is characterized by the weakening of the muscles that are in control of major systems in the human body, resulting in irregular breathing activity during sleep.

3. Consequences of Poor Sleep Due to Allergies

It is important to consider the impact allergies have on sleep to fully address the well-being of the affected. The consequences of poor sleep from allergies do not occur in isolation. Allergies cause sleep to be disrupted by a range of symptoms (i.e., sniffling, itching, sneezing, etc.) which have a variety of implications, including physical issues (i.e., head, chest, and muscle pain) and psychological consequences (i.e., irritability, lack of concentration, and headaches). While this type of outcome is debilitating in itself, psychological disturbances including depression, anxiety, or an overall decrease in well-being underscore the holistic impact of nasal allergens on affected individuals. Approaching sleep qualitatively as an important component within overall wellness stigmatizes those hindered by allergies and poor sleep. The issue at hand is not whether sleep is an important aspect of everyday wellness, but it is the means by which reduced sleep can manifest negative implications for those with chronic or continuous sensitivities to allergens.

Poor quality sleep has wide-reaching and long-term consequences for overall physical health and mental health, creating negative moods and cognitive dysfunctions. Nighttime symptoms of allergies, which are chronic, intermittent, and seasonal, bring further issues into play. The current COVID-19 pandemic has only intensified considerations of sleep quality because of the purported link between weakened immune systems and poor sleep. Although smaller inferences from lost sleep have been made to diseases such as colds and flus, poor sleep quality as a result of poorly managed allergies was not considered in these campaigns, showcasing how the complete picture has not been considered.

3.1. Physical and Mental Health Implications

Hallmarks most commonly associated with poor sleep resulting from allergies include fatigue, daytime sleepiness, irritability, memory and thinking issues, and a general lack of motivation. Common negative health outcomes associated with allergies and poor sleep are memory issues, weight gain or increased appetite with unhealthy metabolic changes, decreased libido, increased infection risk, increased cancer risk, mood changes, and potentially even a higher risk of heart disease and diabetes. Everyone who has ever experienced a restless night fighting off the symptoms of allergies knows that it can have dire physical consequences. Having allergies is simply miserable.

Sleep is often thought to be a critical time in which the mind and body can rest and recharge; an unavoidable aspect of life with equally unavoidable implications. Without rest, bodies operate at a diminished capacity. This can be a liability in terms of both reflexes and mood. We also require sleep to restore physical health and repair tissues. Poor sleep can result in an immune system that operates at a diminished capacity, slowing down recovery from illness and increasing one's susceptibility to infections. As for mental health, sleepiness can dull the ability to concentrate and inhibit problem-solving, and sometimes results in accidents. Studies show an inability to connect emotions with logical responses when we are not getting enough sleep. Active mood swings, anxiety, and irritability have all been associated with inadequate sleep.

Depression and suicide risk are among the most serious effects of ongoing sleep deficiencies.

In the previous section, it was discussed how allergens in the environment can result in a poor night's sleep. Though the impacts may not always seem significant, the consequences of experiencing a low-quality sleep due to allergies can manifest themselves in a variety of ways over time. These consequences may heavily influence a person and destructively impact both their mental and physical health.

4. Creating a Healthy Sleeping Environment

Remove Allergens from the Home: It is possible to have allergens that do not have to be directly in the bedroom at night, but in the house during the day or evening. Cat dander on the underwear of a friend may trigger symptoms when it is in the bedroom and hanging in the bedroom closet. It is important to wash dryer lint screens once or twice a week to reduce cat or dog dander emissions. Dryer vents should never come indoors as these may feed allergens into the home.

Evaluate Ventilation: The sources of allergens in a bedroom are not just the allergens contained in the bedding, mattresses, and pets. Outdoor allergens like pollen and mold can also contaminate the indoor environment through inadequate ventilation of the bedroom area. And most contaminations occur at night, from about 10 p.m. to 4 or 5 a.m., when the outdoors are cooler, bringing allergens inside. "Also, we tend to keep windows open at night to cool down our bedrooms, but this allows more access from outdoors and exposure to allergens," Ramadan says. "Opening windows, especially from 6 p.m. to 8 a.m. when pollen peaks and is counted in the air, brings in much higher amounts of allergens."

Identify Sources: The first step in creating a healthy sleeping environment is identifying what allergens might be present. Dust in pillows, pillow coverings, and the walls may be contaminated with dust mite larvae, known allergens. Similarly, dust and cat or dog dander in pillow coverings, the walls, and on bedroom floors might contribute to allergic rhinitis and worsened airway inflammation in people with asthma. Removing these sources of allergens and minimizing the entry of new allergens helps to prevent unwanted inhaled allergens in the bedroom.

A healthy sleeping environment is key to getting a good night's rest and minimizing the negative impact of allergens. Here are a few strategies for pinpointing and reducing allergens in the bedroom:

4.1. Identifying and Minimizing Allergens in the Bedroom

Other allergens in the bedroom include pets and pet dander or fur. It is recommended to implement a no-pet policy in the sleeping area to prevent allergens from entering the space if someone is allergic to pets. In the case that pets are allowed in the sleeping space, it is advisable to bathe furry pets on a weekly basis and brush them outside the sleeping space. Dust mites can easily make their home in pillows, especially down feathers due to the conducive environment. Washing pillows regularly or using hypoallergenic dust mite-proof pillows can prevent dust mite exposure.

Identifying indoor allergens in the bedroom or sleeping space is crucial for reducing allergic symptoms and creating a high-quality sleeping environment. The mattress can be a big source of dust mites in the bedroom, especially those covered in fabric. It is important to use a mattress cover or protective case over the mattress to prevent dust mite exposure. Additionally, washing linens at high temperatures of 140°F will sanitize linens from dust mites, while also removing other small particles that have accumulated in the bed. If possible, linen and mattresses made of natural fibers or garment-washed linens that are free of formaldehyde and other processing chemicals are recommended.

Modifying the sleeping environment involves several steps. Carpets can be removed in place of hard surface floor covering and washable rugs. The use of quality air filters in the heating and cooling system can help minimize dust, pet dander, and mold. Allergic reaction can be minimized by covering mattresses, pillows, and box springs with protective casings. Sheets and pillowcases should be washed regularly in a hot water setting (i.e., 140°F) to reduce dust mites; this process also sanitizes bedding.

It is important to create a safe, high-quality sleeping environment which is minimally impacted by allergens. The first step is to remove or address the allergen directly. Common sources of allergens in the bedroom include bedding, carpets, and upholstered furniture. Other potential alleged "culprits" include mold and pets.

5. Diet and Lifestyle Changes for Better Sleep

If diet and lifestyle changes are successful, the time it takes to fall asleep and the number of times you wake up during the night may become quicker and fewer, sleep disorders can decrease, and body mass can decrease or stabilize. Individuals who participate in community-based allergy treatments and are educated about the environment, diet, lifestyle, and mind-body changes may be able to manage and prevent sleep disturbance. They may also be able to achieve more rest, work, and everyday activities. Individuals who learn to flourish indoors, where a few are out in the daytime when pollen counts are generally lower, may have even fewer days lost due to disturbed sleep and demonstrated allergy symptoms. Overall, a healthy sleeping environment should use dietary modifications like removing worrying caffeinated elements from your bedtime routine.

It should also be noted that diet plays a role in allergies and sleep in terms of managing discomfort. Eating and avoiding certain foods can result in skin reactions, weight gain, and sinus issues in some individuals. Plant-based diets, which include a rotation of fruits, vegetables, nuts, and seeds, or the Indian Subcontinent "ayurvedic" diet adapted for the West, may lead to fewer allergy symptoms, better sleep, and lower body mass, although these findings are mixed. Additionally, people with mold sensitivities should also avoid coffee, tea, sugar, and mushrooms.

5.1. Impact of Diet on Allergies and Sleep

Indeed, a high-fat diet category that promoted sleep had lower propionate not only in stool but also in breath. These findings suggest that the metabolic effects of diet could have indirect immunologic effects that could influence allergic response and/or sleep. Diet can also have direct metabolic influences on sleep and may trigger sleep disorders such as RLS and snoring. While evidence is growing, more research is needed to determine the direct effects of diet on allergies and sleep. Given that the results of these studies are still inconclusive, it is impossible to predict the exact diet that would promote higher quality sleep in people with allergies in general. Personalized diets are likely the answer, with calculated "immune scores" that could help inform individuals not only of what allergies they may have but also if these allergies are unfavorably introducing sleep loss.

Sleep can be impacted by many outside factors, but perhaps the easiest one to modify is diet. Diet may play a major role in allergies, which have been found to decrease sleep quality. Allergic rhinitis has also been associated with difficulty falling asleep and maintaining sleep, as well as with overall decreased sleep quality. Interestingly, there is emerging data that diet can impact sleep directly, beyond allergies. This is particularly true for components of diet that can be directly stimulating, such as caffeine. In this way, it not only has the potential to change allergies; diet may have the potential to change sleep on an independent level.

6. Allergy Medications and Their Effects on Sleep

Antihistamines address the histamine-induced inflammatory response to allergen particles. Antihistamine medications come in two types: first-generation and second-generation antihistamines. They have a similar mode of action but are grouped by their date of availability. Corticosteroids, or steroids, are drugs used to reduce inflammation in the body. They work by decreasing the inflammation response, leading to less swelling, itching, and other accompanying symptoms. Immunotherapy is a process of re-training an individual's immune system. It works as therapy over time to decrease the allergic response to environmental triggers. These therapies are available in both injections and oral formulations. Decongestants help to decrease swelling in the nasal passages. Immunotherapy is a process of re-training an individual's immune system. It works as therapy over time to decrease the allergic response to environmental triggers. To do this, an individual receives increasing doses of allergens over a period of years until they reach maintenance therapy.

The landscape of treatment options for allergies and the potentially resulting impact on sleep quality is immense and can vary greatly depending on an individual's region of the world, specific health history, and any underlying pre-existing medical conditions that can often be exacerbated by allergies. There are several excellent groups of medications on the market that aim to ease the symptoms of allergies; it is also worth noting that some medications work best with particular forms of allergy triggers. It is important to evaluate available treatments and to decide upon the course of action that works best for a given situation. However, if the presented course of treatment is a medication, it is a very good idea to speak with a healthcare professional about how the medication will impact the body, different potential side effects, and the impact on sleep.

6.1. Types of Allergy Medications

As for the second-generation antihistamines, different determinations have previously been made regarding their influence on sleep. Some investigators have claimed that these agents can impair sleep, while others have issued reports stating that they do not affect sleep. Among the second-generation antihistamines that are frequently used throughout the world, levocetirizine is the only one that has been reported through polysomnography to be associated with impaired sleep. Researchers have not yet reached a consensus regarding the impact of corticosteroid nasal spray, corticosteroid nasal drops, and inhaled corticosteroid use on sleep pattern disturbances. Further studies are necessary to identify the effect of these medications on sleep.

Antihistamines are the most widely used drugs to treat the symptoms of allergies, and they can be separated into first- and second-generation antihistamines. Each type has a distinct impact on sleep. The first-generation antihistamines that make people tired, in particular, are used to treat allergy symptoms and sometimes sleep disorders such as non-24-hour sleep-wake disorders. As such, first-generation antihistamines can alleviate symptoms of both allergies and insomnia. However, although first-generation antihistamines can improve symptoms, they have also been reported to impair sleep maintenance and sleep architecture. A previous study reported that these drugs can increase the number of arousals during sleep in particular. Therefore, they are not always used in combination with this purpose.

7. Non-Pharmacological Interventions for Allergy-Induced Sleep Issues

7.2. Humidifiers A viable alternative to air purifiers, humidifiers increase the relative humidity of an environment while reducing indoor air pollution. One study showed that when comparing air purifiers with cool mist humidifiers and control in air purifier users, a significant reduction in allergen symptoms and better sleep was attained with the cool air mist humidifier. Overall, more than 85% of participants in the study agreed that the cool mist had improved the management of their asthma and allergies.

7.1. Air purifiers Air purifiers - either HEPA or activated charcoal - may reduce inhaled allergen levels. A study has shown that both activated charcoal and HEPA filters have significantly increased melatonin levels and have reduced daytime sleepiness, RMSA, and the concentration of the exhaled nitric oxide in patients with allergic rhinitis. HEPA filters, however, can disrupt sleep through an increase in acoustic disturbance if the bedroom is small enough. The use of an activated charcoal filter and not HEPA filter has been shown to ameliorate pet allergen load, interleukin 6 and disturbed sleep, in boys with allergic rhinitis during a pet in-home challenge. These findings have led to the notion that a factor contributing to the poor sleep in allergic individuals is exposure to secondary irritant pollutants rather than a direct allergic reaction.

Non-pharmacological interventions

Humidifiers: Similar to air purifiers, the main goal of humidifiers is to create an advantageous environment through increased humidity, as it has been shown to impede the spread of airborne pathogens in residential environments. More specifically, humidification can reduce dust and dust mites as well as mold in the home. Despite the advantages, selecting the right type of system is exceptionally important, as overuse can cause other problems, such as rapidly accelerating mold growth. Overall, central humidifiers are considered the most effective option for overall comfort, while vaporizers and air conditioners are also beneficial. Another consideration is the option to choose a system that comes equipped with an antibacterial filter for improved sleep hygiene and health. In addition to these, common non-pharmacological interventions will be described in greater detail to provide specific guidance for managing conditions known to cause poor sleep.

Air purifiers: Most air purifiers contain a mechanical filter with a high efficiency rate. A high-efficiency particulate air filter can remove 99.97% of airborne particles larger than 0.3 mm, while an ultra-low particulate air filter is actually better for many allergens because it can remove particles as small as 0.1 mm. However, some purifiers come with a high-quality filter upgrade that may be required for the best results. In addition to mechanical filters, many purifiers contain a physical barrier (ionizer, dry charged plates) or chemical additives (reactive oxygen species, hydroxyl radicals, or ozone). However, chemical additives tend to be less useful for allergies. Regardless of the type of filter, sizing of the air purifier is the most crucial component in the decision-making process. Therefore, it is essential to determine the size of both the room where the purifier will be used and the overall space for reliable performance. Further, with the constant updates and new models and types available on the market, coupling with additional product research before purchasing is recommended to ensure the best results.

8. Cognitive Behavioral Therapy for Insomnia (CBT-I) and Allergies

This novel study explicitly described the link between allergic rhinitis and insomnia. It also described the importance of allergies to the participant group in distress following difficulty falling asleep, staying asleep, and resuming sleep should the participant wake during the night. As discussed above, sleep could be a point of intervention through decreasing morning impairments in cognitive function, work or social limitations due to anxiety, irritability, fatigue, and struggling to find the energy to engage in social activities. From current research on the management of allergic rhinitis and its accompanying phenomena, it is suggestive of the importance of targeting sleep in the context of allergic rhinitis. Implications and future research are discussed.

There is minimal literature evaluating the impact of CBT-I in the context of allergies exclusively. In a 2018 review examining the impact of sleep hygiene behaviors in allergic rhinitis, five out of six studies (observational N=1; interventional N=5) noted significant sleep disturbances resulting from allergies. However, two studies also noted improvements in sleep following initiation of antihistamine treatment. As such, many of the health problems that may be relieved through environmental control are, in essence, sleep problems. Exclusively, antidepressants, anticonvulsants, and hypnotics, among the classes of medications outlined by ISAH, have been investigated in patients with allergies. In the context of allergy, CBT-I might be a particularly palatable non-pharmacological intervention for sleep. Participants in this review engaged in CBT-I presented by a GP or given self-directed workbooks. Pharmaceutical treatment of insomnia was not discussed. As such, this is the first study that directly evaluated the utility of any non-pharmacologic treatment when experiencing allergic rhinitis.

Changing thoughts on insomnia: The role of CBT-I in the context of allergies

8.1. Benefits of CBT-I for Allergy Sufferers

Why the focus on cognitive function and sleep? To elaborate, the current version of the thinking concerning the interaction of allergic disease, cognitive function, sleep, inflammation, and the immune system is that their interaction is complex and multifaceted. This review does not seek to explore the immune and inflammatory specifics of the interaction between allergic disease and sleep but rather it focuses on the main guiding factors to sleep disruptions arising from allergic diseases within the context of primary insomnia as defined. CBT-I views sleep also from a position of a number of interlocking processes that maintain adequate sleep. Width of the home to cover the 8.1. a. Personalized Implementation of CBT-I for Allergy Sufferers. An important adjunct of CBT-I involves helping individuals maintain a 'clean and attractive sleep environment' from engaging in individual instrumental behavioral change through to making decisions concerning the maintenance of the home environment.

What do we offer in this particular subheading? Insomnias associated with allergy are particularly poignant, resulting in individualized factors affecting sleep. There is the likelihood that patients may also report problems with entrenched insomnia, which is the focus of this narrative review. Hence, allergic diseases do not exist in isolation; they operate in the context of an interaction of patients with a complex multi-faceted system. Cognitive-behavioral therapy for insomnia (CBT-I) takes this broad contextual view. This lends itself particularly well to treating the sleep disruptions of those with allergic diseases as a starting point, addressing not the allergic disease directly but the perceived sleep disruption falling under the insomnia construct.

9. Conclusion and Future Directions

Insomnia is the syndrome we currently know most about: it is bidirectionally related to allergic disorders; it responds well to, among other things, cognitive-behavioral therapy; and it is well-documented to be comorbid with other psychological disorders. A bidirectional link suggests that treatment with sleep aids should improve both syndromes, and this is what is observed empirically. It is possible that similar research will reveal that nasally-bronchially mediated stuffiness and cough will also respond well to clinical trials with multi-modality evidence-based therapies (e.g. for respiratory treatment; g. antihistamines, possibly montelukast, and oral corticosteroids administered along with treatment targeting associated factors such as obesity). Given the continuous demands of life in the 21st century, these studies underscore the importance of learning as much as we can about how to create residential habitats that foster the very best for rest, recuperation, and rejuvenation.

A complete understanding of how allergies impact sleep is limited by the dearth of research on this topic. The strongest evidence we have suggests that allergies can incite sleep-disordered breathing and symptomatic complaints about sleep quality. While not reviewed here, there is a veritable mountain of research suggesting that more fragmented sleep can have a "daytime" carrying-over negative impact on cognitive functioning and wellbeing. Decongesting nasal passageways and using HEPA filters will cut down on allergen and particulate "dose" during the night; however, it is not entirely clear if doing so will improve sleep quality or mediate allergic complaints during the day for all people.

9.1. Summary of Key Findings

Collecting new knowledge on factors that contribute to chronic disease, such as the interaction of allergens with sleep, is crucial for our society. Moving forward, efforts need to be made to put these findings to the test, improving on them, and disseminating them. Thanks to the internet, we are already capable of applying these principles in our practices. We hope to be able to investigate further the effects of environmental control on other conditions such as chronic sinusitis and obesity. According to the American Academy of Allergy and Immunology, allergies are the 5th leading cause of chronic diseases in the United States. In 2000, Americans made 11.1 million visits to physicians' offices for allergic rhinitis, and the direct costs of these visits in 1996 would have been $250 million in 1996 USD. In a 1997 telephone survey of 1001 participants, 19% of Americans reported having chronic insomnia, and among these respondents, 92% also had allergies. Research including the assessment of sleep hygiene in the home environment can benefit these patients, while also addressing additional risks of allergen exposure. Other examples of these benefits appear ahead in this essay. In order to assess the environmental control information currently disseminated, this author undertook an initial investigation of commercial messages regarding products marketed to reduce allergens. This author was interested in whether the ideal message we uncovered last year is being disseminated, and whether it has been validated with current scientific methods. Results of this study are included ahead. Avoiding exposure to allergens is one of the many practices used to deal with allergies. This essay describes some of the research currently available regarding allergen control in the environment. Regulatory agencies produce guides for the use of other agencies to provide guidance on allergenic airborne agents and allergens, and other documents benchmarking allergens in indoor environments. These treatments have made significant progress towards removing allergens from the indoor environment.

The objective of this essay was to assess the impact of allergies on quality of sleep, as well as to consider the strategies available to those seeking to establish environments for sleep that are free of allergens. Techniques used to accomplish this include a review of the literature relating to allergenic abatement, an investigation of the marketing consumers typically encounter regarding these devices. Findings include that cetirizine and fexofenadine are both likely more effective in lessening allergic symptoms than diphenhydramine is, and that some vacuum cleaners equipped with HEPA filtration systems are capable of removing allergens from household flooring. Washable vacuum bags for such a device seem not to lead to allergen re-contamination in the air. Air purifiers capable of serving to reduce allergen levels can be effective for the consumer. It is likely unnecessary to have a HEPA filter in the indoor environmental control plan of a person who is managing asthma in a single room. Covering pillows has been shown to be superior to putting them in allergenic covers. Allergenic commercially marketed stuffed toys were found to be no less likely to retain their contents than unstuffed toys were. Fumigation with acaricides may lead to improvements in the asthmatic conditions of sensitive individuals. Also, extensive mite abatement measures are often less effective than those that are less rigorous.

9 7 9 8 8 5 9 9 4 3 8 6 9